Your Amazing Itty Bitty® Self-Care for Caregivers Book

15 Key Steps to Building a
Care for You Action Plan

Janie Becker, CMT,
the Encourager

Published by Itty Bitty® Publishing
A subsidiary of S & P Productions, Inc.

Printed in the United States of America

Itty Bitty Publishing
311 Main Street, Suite D
El Segundo, CA 90245
(310) 640-8885

ISBN: 978-1-950326-12-9

The Importance of Self-Care for Caregivers

15 Key Steps to Building a Care for You Action Plan

You want your loved ones to feel cared for and safe through the aging process. You know it's important for them to be at home if possible. As important as it is for them to be cared for, it is equally vital for you to be cared for. The purpose of this self-care book is to help you create your 15-step action plan toward relevant self-care. In this Itty Bitty ® book, Janie Becker identifies the obstacles caregivers experience and shows creative, productive ways to overcome overwhelm and emotional exhaustion.

In this book you will learn:

- How to listen to your inner voice
- How to give yourself permission for self-care
- How to create balance for harmony
- Where to find support and resources

If you have been putting off your own self-care to provide care for others, it's time to take a moment for yourself and read this book today!

Dedication Page

This Itty Bitty® book is dedicated to my precious sisters, Sue Ann Becker Chicots and Mary Jo Becker Rowe. They were brilliant and dependable helpmates who I counted on for ideas, solutions, support, respite help, physical labor to move households, help making critical care and end-of-life decisions during nine years of elder care for four elders. Their guidance in writing letters and scripts for talking to hospital administrators, nursing directors, doctors, case managers, social workers, and caring support strategies for our parents and family elders was exemplary.

I am forever grateful for their guidance, support, and encouragement, and pray you will find this book useful for your caregiving situation.

Stop by our Itty Bitty® website to find
interesting blog entries regarding …

www.IttyBittyPublishing.com

Or visit Janie Becker at:

https://www.lessbrainstressnow.com

Table of Contents

Introduction

The purpose of this Itty Bitty® self-care book
is to help you create your 15-step action plan
toward relevant self-care. Janie has helped
clients identify the obstacles to self-care and
create productive ways to overcome
overwhelm. Help is available whether you are
paid full-time, part-time, as an unpaid
volunteer caregiver, or provide support from
far away.

This book will supply information to assist
you in starting to take care of yourself today
while you keep up your caregiving mission.
You may want to gift this book to a friend
who needs help to focus on their own self-
care.

Blessings to all who CARE with:
        Compassion
        Attention
        Respect
        Encouragement

"Self-care is not selfish. You cannot serve
from an empty vessel." *Eleanor Brown*

Step 1
Permission

Many caregivers put everyone else before they think of themselves. Whether you are a volunteer caregiver or are paid to care for someone else, you must give yourself permission to take care of YOU first.

1. Caregiving is hard work physically and emotionally. It becomes more challenging when you have no warning of it coming and you put your own life aside to care for aging parents, a sibling, friend, or neighbor.
2. You can lose your own life when you neglect yourself and your own needs.
3. You deserve to take good care of yourself and protect your health.
4. Your attitude that self-care is important sets your mind in the mode that it is OK and even makes it OK for others to accept.
5. Caring for yourself can change the quality of your life and those for whom you provide care.

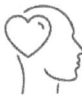

1

Give Yourself Permission

- Give yourself permission to take care of yourself.
- Affirmation: "It's OK to give myself permission to take care of myself today."
- Plan time for yourself on the calendar.
- Access examples of caregivers who successfully care for themselves.
- Make a list of who you know that is caring for their parents successfully. Ask them for tips and ideas.
- Go to www.lessbrainstressnow.com for resources, free monthly Caregivers Corner newsletter, and free caregiver e-book.
- Boundaries—tell others this is *My Time*.
- List reasons why this permission is important to you and keep reminders for reference.
- Scientific research supports the importance of self-care. Caregiver expert websites: Dr Daniel Amen, MD; AARP Caregiver; Dave Nassaney; Sher Berk.

Step 2
Signs You've Lost Your Self

Overwhelm can come when you have no plan or your to-do list is waylaid by emergencies, unplanned illness, piles of paperwork like medical bills, incessant telephone calls, unnecessary interruptions, and too much to do on top of the daily hygiene care for your aging parents, cooking, cleaning, laundry, and so much more.

1. You know the needs of your mom and/or your dad (whomever you are caring for) better than your own.
2. You feel time and energy are out of control.
3. You're unable to keep a regular schedule.
4. You say to yourself, "I'll get back to my own stuff some day" (exercise, personal needs, housework, projects, paying the bills timely).
5. You feel like all you do is work, chores, medical appointments, pharmacy, government agencies. There is no time to do something for you.
6. You can't think straight; feeling stuck.

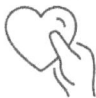

Signs You've Lost Your Self-Recover

- Who are you? Where did the real you go? Spend five minutes every morning to check in to ask, **"What can I do today to take good care of myself?"** For ideas and suggestions, go to www.lessbrainstressnow.com and visit the resources page.
- Since you calendar appointments for their care, schedule five minutes in your planner or Smartphone in the morning and the evening to do something for YOU and make it your priority.
- Put the most important personal project on the to-do list, something that you can do while being the "caree's" companion, such as when you're waiting in the doctor's office or they are watching TV, napping, or otherwise preoccupied and don't need supervision.
- Identify one task of the project that can be done in 5-10 minutes. You've heard the expression, "You can eat an elephant one bite at a time." Break the project into small chunks, which will allow you to do the parts in sequence toward eventual completion.

Step 3
Neglect of Your Self

Caregivers typically sacrifice their own needs for the needs of others, to the point of exhaustion, anger, resentment, chronic scowling, rude remarks and secret feelings of guilt.

What creates neglect? Constant denial or inattention to your own needs, fears, sorrow, physical, emotional, and spiritual depletion.

1. Sacrifice of your own routine can lead to physical problems such as headaches, dehydration, stress, weight gain, hair loss, nervous tic, distraction, or lack of focus.
2. Neglect of your own self-care impacts others. By scheduling your own self-care like quiet time, walks, your favorite workout time, half-hour breaks to do a hobby, or visits with friends can set an example of healing choices and create space for health.
3. Neglect of your own health may risk alienating friends and important people.
4. Create consistent space for your self-care, to increase your confidence, ability to remain strong, healthy, and joyful.

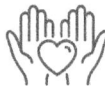

Tips to Overcome Neglect

Take ten minutes to think about what your life would be like if you had more time to yourself to do what you love or what is most important to you.

- Take a pack of index cards.
- List one task, activity, idea, hobby on each card with a time estimate for each task. List steps to completion.
- Prioritize each card in pencil with how important and fulfilling the task or activity is to you on a scale of 1-10 (1 is low priority, 10 is high priority or importance.)

Now, look at next week on the calendar and schedule one task each day at a specific time.

- List any items or supplies you need for each task or activity on the back of the index card for each one.
- Create a shopping list for the dollar store or an inexpensive source (supplies closet) to gather the items you need.
- Gather a tote for the items. Store in a special place you can access easily. Organize it. Schedule your time.

Step 4
Listen to Your Inner Voice

Have you heard the phrase, *Listen for that still small inner voice?* Have you ever been led to do something but didn't know why, you did it anyway and it worked out well for you?

The chaos around you can get intense with the tasks of caregiving and listening for others' needs—jumping every time the phone rings until you know who is calling, handling unexpected medical and emotional needs, and adapting to constant changes in physical demands. Knowing the difference between whether each need is important, urgent, an emergency, or crisis is critical for your own care.

1. Stop a moment and listen to that inner voice, get a clear message, or consult with an expert, or a reliable, supportive friend.
2. If many options are revealed, make a list of them and use the T chart method to determine pros and cons of each to help reveal the best option for the circumstance.
3. Meditation practice can help develop your ability to listen to that inner voice.

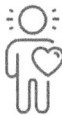

Access Your Inner Voice

Many meditation methods are available.

- Hypnotherapy specialists can guide you, and are accessible, through the Itty Bitty® website authors and publisher.
- Meditation CDs are available at your local library or bookstore, and coaches can be found at the holistic chamber of commerce in your area.

Senior centers and community colleges offer classes for yoga, meditation, tai chi chih and more gentle methods to calm your spirit and reduce the anxiety in your mind.

- Affirmations and positive thoughts are useful tools you can learn from teachers and tools (Caregivers Corner newsletter).
- Lavender essential oil is especially useful diffused or applied to your wrists, back of your neck and soles of your feet before bedtime or during healing sessions.

Step 5
Do Something

Often elder caregivers forget how important it is to have a self-care plan for their health and safety. Ask yourself, what is my self-care plan? Have I written it down and set it into action? If so, great! If not, let's start here to create your self-care plan. Follow the steps below.

1. Take the index cards from Step 3. Review them and decide the top ten activities that you feel are most important to create your plan.
2. The most important element of this step is to DO SOMETHING, ONE THING. TAKE ACTION. This will give you a sense of getting movement and as you do the next important thing, big or small, you will gain momentum and a little excitement to keep taking action on your plan. You are worth the time investment!

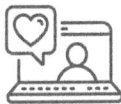

Do Something

You've heard the saying, "You must start to finish," or, "The longest journey begins with the first step."

- Take your plan and list the steps.
- Prioritize the steps.
- Start the first step. If it's too big, break it down into smaller steps.

Acknowledge yourself for starting. Each time you do one of the steps in your plan, you'll be closer to accepting that you deserve to take care of yourself. As you feel stronger and more active, you will set the environment for others to accept that you deserve the time to be active for yourself. Track your activities and rate how you feel upon completion. Celebrate each time you do movement or activity. Even ten minutes of movement counts.

Step 6
Breathing Techniques

Our bodies breathe automatically through the autonomic system unless we're under physical or emotional stress. As the pressure increases when we're overwhelmed, we may hold our breath (shallow breath) or hyperventilate (breathe too fast and start to get dizzy). You can learn many simple techniques to protect yourself from injury and harm. Here are a few methods to practice:

1. Yoga breathing: breathe out, breathe in, and hold it for the count of four. Repeat as you stretch your arms out and upward.
2. Andrew Weil, MD breathing technique: breathe in to the count of six, hold for the count of six, and exhale to the count of six. Repeat three times.
3. Relaxation response technique: can reduce stress symptoms. Pick a focus word. Sit comfortably, relaxing from head to toes. Focus on your breath in and out. Allow thoughts to pass.
4. Tai Chi Chih: breathe in and raise your arms; start with a rocking motion and learn about alignment, circularity, polarity, softness, and more.

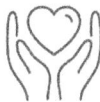

Breathing Tips and Techniques

Most caregivers breathe 17,000 breaths a day.

- Awareness breath involves feeling the in breath and the exhale and becoming aware of the change in your body.
- Breathe slowly in through the nose, out through the mouth.
- Awareness breathing can relax your body or increase your energy.
- Breathe deeply before activity/exercise.

Using essential oils as you breathe may enhance the effects of your breathing techniques.

- Sacred Frankincense™ may enhance your breathing exercise.
- Northern Lights Black Spruce comes from British Columbia, Canada and its invigorating scent may create a fresh aromatic atmosphere during your meditation.

Step 7
Balance to Harmony

Many caregivers have expressed that they want to end the overwhelm they feel and find balance in their lives. Balance is different for each caregiver. When you feel off-balance, unable to focus, unable to keep on task due to constant interruptions and unforeseen obstacles, the best way to respond is to follow your plan step-by-step, even when the next step is to stop, rest and regroup.

1. Identify what balance looks like to you.
2. List three key steps to follow to feel more balanced.
3. Complete the first step and notice how you feel. Proceed to the next step and acknowledge your progress. After the third step, check again to see how balanced you feel.
4. Revise your plan if you need to do so. Many caregivers find it helpful to make small changes for the right balance each week as circumstances change.
5. Allowing others to help with tasks can lift some of the pressure you feel.
6. Write feelings in your journal.
7. Diffuse or use Peace & Calming® essential oil to set your environment.

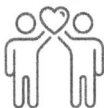

Balance to Harmony

Now that you've established a sense of balance, what will it be like when you feel harmony with your environment and your goals?

- One meaning of harmony is agreement or accord, unity or cooperation. Decide what harmony looks like for your circumstance.
- Some caregivers experience harmony by following a clear self-care plan with the synchronicity of support, respite care, and improving healthy lifestyle choices.
- Consider making a drop of Harmony™ essential oil part of your self-care plan for calming and grounding.

Step 8
MOVE

Hundreds of scientists and kinesiologists have studied the positive outcomes of physical movement on relieving chronic diseases and stress.

1. Physical movement can range from a stretching routine, walking, running, weight training, dancing, Zumba class, exercise machines, and more.
2. Even imagining physical activity can have a positive effect on your body, mind and spirit connection.
3. Positive thoughts based on a belief that you have the time and energy to move easily and frequently can reduce stress.
4. As you improve your ability to imagine positive movement, you can improve your willingness to be more active with a definite daily plan.

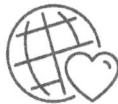

More on Movement

Movement can help you, the caregiver, reduce the anxiety and stress you feel.

- Ten minutes of stair climbing or intense stationary bicycling can speed your metabolism which may reduce your blood pressure and frequency of headaches, neck, and shoulder strain.
- Thirty to sixty minutes of aquafit in the pool can help increase joint mobility, muscle tone, and improve your sleep.

Physiologists have shown us that even ten-minute spurts of activity a few times a day can help us feel clearer in our thinking and making choices. A variety of movement activities can help you breathe better and reduce anxiety symptoms. Here are a few ideas.

- Marching steps (high knees) – 5 minutes; stand up, sit down – 2x to start
- Calf lifts – 10x; Toe raises – 10 repetitions
- Climb steps for 5 minutes, up and down (hold railing with care)
- Breathe in and raise arms as far as comfortable 3x; bend at hips and touch toes 3x. Add more reps as you improve.

Step 9
Sleep

You can incorporate simple techniques to increase the time you dedicate to sleep and the quality of your daily sleep.

1. Use darkening drapes to keep light out of your bedroom or sleeping area.
2. Limit or eliminate high magnetic field devices in your bedroom (TV, radio, cellphone, high wires).
3. Stop water intake at 6 or 8 pm (to reduce number of bladder calls in the middle of the night).
4. If your sleeping partner(s) (person or pet) snores too loudly or too much and ear plugs don't block the noise, consider sleeping in a separate room.
5. Consider a white noise machine or wave sound machine. Some insomniacs use these devices to increase sound sleep.

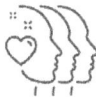

More Sleep Tips

Doctors, therapists, and sleep technicians have reported how important sufficient daily sleep is for a healthy lifestyle.

You can incorporate simple techniques to increase the time you dedicate to sleep and the quality of your daily sleep.

- Do gentle yoga or movement ten minutes after your bathing and teeth brushing routine before bedtime.
- Go to bed at the same time and arise at the same time every day as much as you can. It takes a few weeks for your body to make this a reliable habit.
- When you awake too soon, get up and read or write in your journal, until you get sleepy and return to your bed or do some light stretching or meditation.

Step 10
Support

What does support look like for your caregiving situation? Have you included respite care from other family members, friends, neighbors, or paid caregivers who can provide help for your caregiving situation in your self-care plan?

Here are a few ideas to consider for the support section of your plan:

1. Positive focused caregiver support groups.
2. Regular family meetings - check in to share how members can provide help.
3. Daily adult care in the neighborhood.
4. Talk with doctors and nurses who care for your elders to get ideas for their care and your self-care.

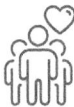

More Support Techniques

Research adult day care options.

- Find out about daily availability, costs, staffing, activities with local adult care facilities.
- Research options with geriatric specialists.
- Check with your neighbors and friends of your parents.
- Keep care kit and medical history information handy for respite caregivers with emergency contact numbers.
- Talk with parents' neighbors and friends to determine whether they are willing and able to help you; give them regular updates and cautions.
- Share the checklist of what to do when respite caregivers are available to help.

Step 11
FUN

Can you identify what adding fun to your lifestyle would look like? What would it feel like to feel joyful every day you wake up, ready for a smooth easy caregiving day?

1. Include in your card deck simple ideas for your dedicated self-care fun time.
2. What is the most fun you remember as a kid? Is it something you can include in your daily routine for ten minutes or more?
3. Do you have a friend or family member who always sees the funny side of things? Plan to talk with them regularly and get their support.
4. Listening to giggling babies and toddlers can lighten the stress and sadness you may feel sometimes.
5. Learn to laugh at any mistakes or mishaps. It is said we make ten a day. Allow yourself forgiveness.

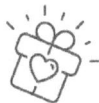

More Fun Ideas

How important is incorporating fun into your self-care plan? AARP social workers and therapists give workshops locally to provide resources and ideas for adding fun to your self-care plan to lighten the stress and avoid burnout.

- Comedy clubs
- Comedian websites, Laugh Factory
- YouTube funny animal videos
- Daily Laughs website
- Silly health cartoons
- Readers Digest inspiring stories
- Write the best thing that happened in your journal every day. Review it occasionally and praise your source.

Step 12
Feelings and Emotions

Ignoring your feelings can create even more anxiety and physical distress. Acknowledge your feelings as much as you can as close to the time you have the emotions of sadness, grief, joy, depression.

1. Write in your journal the situations of the day and your feelings. Great release can come from putting the pen to your journal.
2. Share your feelings with a support group.
3. Keep a daily 1 (low) to 10 (great) scale of feelings on your calendar. Notice at the end of the month how many numbers over seven scores you wrote down.
4. Schedule respite care with trusted caregivers on call or regular times in the week.
5. Determine the best essential oils to have handy for keeping yourself calm and clear in mind. Tranquil™ Roll-On is one of my favorites. Sign up for the monthly Caregivers Corner newsletter for suggestions and tips.
www.lessbrainstressnow.com

Tips About Feelings and Emotions

Medical professionals advise caregivers to take care of yourself by daily exercise, healthy food choices, and help from support to avoid chronic illness. You've heard about the increase of pheromones when you move and keep active.

- Hydrating your body with water every hour keeps your brain healthy.
- Ensure you eat more protein and foods with zinc to maintain your calm patience.
- Share how you feel with a reliable friend or therapist.
- Listen to your still small voice to know what choices are best for you.
- Consistently keep movement in your self-care plan to ensure body, mind, and spirit strength.
- Check with your doctor or acupuncturist for support supplements to keep consistent health focus.

Step 13
Healthy Brain Foods

Numerous medical doctors, nutritionists and dietitians recommend balanced nutrition and frequent hydration to maintain optimal health. The U.S. Nuclear Regulatory Commission lists two categories of radiation exposure:

1. Natural resources - cosmic (air travel), terrestrial (soil), internal (5%).
2. Manmade resources - industrial and occupational, medical procedures and nuclear medicine.

Foods for thought and a healthy brain.

1. Sufficient protein is integral for clarity of mind and strength of body from plants like edamame, quinoa, nuts, lentils, beans.
2. A balance of carbohydrates, fats, vitamins and amino acids keeps healthy caregivers able to make clear decisions.
3. Green leafy vegetables like spinach, kale, broccoli, romaine lettuce, and mushrooms provide protein, vitamins, and minerals.
4. Combat radiation with brazil nuts, seaweed, parsley, cilantro, and fermented foods. Know the source for safety.

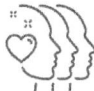

More About Healthy Brain Foods

Many fruits and vegetables can provide you with good fiber, fat, and protein to maintain healthy brain function and stamina for those challenging, high-stress days.

- Raspberries, blackberries, figs, and pears rate highest for antioxidants and vitamins.
- Artichokes, peas, okra, acorn squash, and Brussels sprouts are recommended as vitamin and mineral rich.
- Black beans, legumes, chickpeas, split peas, and legumes rate high for protein and minerals.
- Walnuts, almonds, chia and flax seeds, and quinoa are highest in minerals and protein for healthy brain function.
- Source: Doctor Josh Axe, DNM, DC, CNS

Step 14
Good *Vibrations*

You may be aware that everything has a frequency. When humans are healthy, our vibration is high. When we're ill, our vibration is low. Sound healing is a great tool for good health.

Many of us get distracted with our caregiving responsibilities regardless of good intentions. Here are a few tips to help you easily add to your frequency.

1. Studies show geriatricians use musical techniques to boost mental acuity.
2. Musicologists have helped sufferers of chronic neurological disease increase their cognitive skills with singing along with familiar songs and hymns.
3. Some physicians sing songs during exams of frightened or confused patients to help them relax, and recommend their caregivers play favorite types of music.
4. One of our caregiver clients uses a favorite jazz station with familiar tunes from the 1940s, 50s, and 60s for their elder clients and reports it helps reduce her own stress and keeps her joyful when making meals and doing daily hygiene chores for her care recipient.

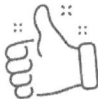

Good *Vibrations*

Another proven popular method to maintain our healthy vibration is to use pure and potent essential oils.

- A favorite universal essential oil for keeping positive focus as a caregiver is peppermint, known for an aroma that promotes feelings of peace and calm, supporting digestive, mental and respiratory health.
- Roman chamomile has a sweet, herbaceous aroma that can help create a calming effect, especially useful for feelings of anxiety and worry.

There is also a yoga hand technique many caregivers find useful to lower stress levels while dealing with all the daily issues that can heighten the feelings of overwhelm.

For more detailed information, go to
https://www.lessbrainstressnow.com
and contact Janie for more information.

Step 15
Real Solutions for Self-Care

What does self-care mean to you? By giving yourself permission to make time for your plan, you can schedule time to breathe and stretch every day and do one thing. Do first things first after you identify your priorities for your-SELF.

1. Identify who can help you with support to create balance and clarity for you.
2. Use your task cards to plan your self-care on your calendar.
3. Meditate every day. Start with five minutes of quiet and focus on your breath.
4. Use positive affirmations and thoughts.
5. Stretch and move.
6. Eat healthy and drink lots of water.
7. Laugh and be joyful.

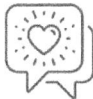

Real Solutions for Self-Care

Track your progress in your journal each week.

- Check in with your support system often.
- Update or revise your task cards monthly.
- Find a quiet time and space to focus and breathe. Access meditation sources for practice.
- Create your own affirmations or use the affirmations in the monthly Caregivers Corner newsletter at https://www.lessbrainstressnow.com
- Choose a movement activity. Do it at least ten minutes each day. Add more minutes as you can make time.
- Choose healthy proteins, fresh vegetables, and fruits in season.
- Remember, water helps reduce stress, anxiety, and depression.
- Find reasons to laugh and use Joy™ essential oil to lighten your spirit and promote a positive outlook.

You've finished. Before you go ...

Tweet/share that you finished this book.

Please star rate this book.

Reviews are solid gold to writers. Please take a few minutes to give us some itty bitty feedback at Amazon Kindle.

32

ABOUT THE AUTHOR

Janie Becker, Certified Massage Therapist (CMT), the Encourager, served as an expected volunteer elder caregiver for four elders over nine years, learning to adapt and choose the best options for her Father, Step-Mom, Aunt and Uncle. During this journey she often felt the spectrum of emotions from I-can-do-this to exhaustion and overwhelm. With the help of two loving sisters, numerous health professionals at the Veterans' Administration and SCAN healthcare staff, steady faith, supportive friends and the guidance of an excellent geriatric social worker, Janie gathered resources and ways to reframe the circumstances for the family to keep the health, finances, and dignity of their elders through the aging process.

She works with caregiving clients to find positive options for time and energy self-care solutions. She will consult with you and your family to help ease the maze of overwhelm. She offers a variety of healing techniques and massage services. She speaks before nursing associations, care facilities, geriatric physicians, and other groups to share healthy caregiving tips.

Janie conducts monthly educational workshops in Long Beach, CA, USA. The monthly Caregivers Corner newsletter is available by visiting the website: https://www.lessbrainstressnow.com

If you enjoyed this Itty Bitty® Book you might also like…

- **Your Amazing Itty Bitty® Affirmations Book, 15 Ways to Make Empowering Messages Work for You** – Micaela Passeri

- **Your Amazing Itty Bitty® Self-Esteem Book** – Jade Elizabeth

- **Your Amazing Itty Bitty® Eldercare Book** – John S. Smith, Jr., RN

Or many more relevant Itty Bitty® books available online at www.ittybittypublishing.com.

www.ingramcontent.com/pod-product-compliance
Lightning Source LLC
Chambersburg PA
CBHW060659280326
41933CB00012B/2245